Anti-Inflamm
Critical Tips a
How to Eat Healthy and
Prevent Inflammation

Food Rules for the Anti-Inflammation Diet

By: Robert Wilson

TABLE OF CONTENTS

Robert Wilson
PUBLISHERS NOTES

DEDICATION

This book is dedicated to my aunt Maria who battles with inflammation every day.

Robert Wilson

Chapter 1 - What Is the Anti-Inflammatory Diet and What Damage Does It Cause?

Inflammation is what happens when the body responds to injury, but sometimes person gets a type of inflammation in the body that causes various illnesses like cancer, heart problems or diabetes. But some people believe inflammation can be countered through an anti-inflammatory diet, which is similar to a Mediterranean diet and eating style.

What Makes Someone Get Chronic Inflammation in the Body?

Being overweight can contribute to there being too much inflammation in the body. It causes infection and disease that then causes problems with sugar regulation and so the person gains weight. Then, the body continues on into a pattern that is hard to stop and even more inflammation occurs. Foods eaten today by many people don't help, as a diet of processed food, saturated fat products, fried foods, refined sugars and trans fats makes even more inflammation to occur in the body.

If you want to avoid contributing to the process, you have to get rid of these foods in your diet. That means you can't eat things like white bread or crackers, potato chips, fast foods, processed luncheon meats, margarine, high fructose corn syrup, high fat cheese, sugar, and vegetable shortening products.

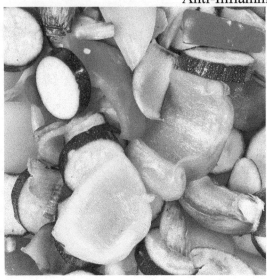

So, What Can You Eat?

If you want to take on an anti-inflammatory diet to help get rid of this cycle of inflammation in the body, you have to start eating certain kinds of foods and introducing certain lifestyle changes. Foods such as omega-3 fatty acids (i.e. fish, walnuts, and flaxseed, etcup) help, along with lean meat, soybeans, tofu, nuts, whole grains, fresh fruits, veggies, legumes, beans, and certain kinds of herbs or spices like garlic, chili pepper, turmeric, basil, ginger, red pepper, cinnamon, cayenne, oregano, and paprika to help give your foods some flavor. You should also drink green, oolong or white tea and red wine is also ok to drink.

To follow the Anti-Inflammatory Diet you need to eat nine servings a day of fruit and veggies, especially those with vitamin A, C, E and beta carotene. Plus oils like olive and canola are good. Lean meats can include poultry, and certain kinds of seafood like cold water fish like sardines and salmon. Eggs with added omega 3s are ok, as well as seeds, and avocados. You can also eat dark chocolate for a treat.

Robert Wilson

Cultures that are known to eat like this have been studied to show they have less disease and inflammation in their bodies. However, some of these diseases are also due to aging and can bring pain and suffering to people as they get older. Plus, other factors like smoking, drinking excessive alcohol, auto immune issues or genetics can also play a factor in causing bodily problems like inflammation.

Benefits of the Anti-Inflammatory Diet

The Anti-Inflammatory diet is touted to some degree by the American Heart Association since they say you should have a diet rich in these types of foods to prevent heart disease. It may also help to prevent problems like Alzheimer's and cancers. It may also help with lowering bad LDL cholesterol in the body. In this diet people should eat half their calories from carbohydrates, about 30 percent of their foods should be fats, and about 30 percent of the foods should be proteins. The diet also provides a goodly amount of fiber, with at least 23 grams a day in a sample menu, whereas the government guidelines say we should get 22 to 34 grams a day.

The diet also has the advantage of making people not feeling hungry and gives a high feeling of being full and satisfied, possibly due to the high amounts of fiber.

Things to consume to best follow the anti-inflammatory diet

Omega-3 fatty acids – Comes from things like fish oil, flaxseed powder, raw nuts, and certain oils like sesame or canola.

Quercetin – This ingredient is present in foods like grapes, onion, garlic, apples, and broccoli.

Resveratrol - This ingredient is present in red wine, which is promoted as drinking a glass or two a day on the anti-inflammatory diet.

Polyphenols – This ingredient is found in things like blueberries or blackberries, as well as cranberries.

Antioxidants – This ingredient is found in things like green or red peppers, tomatoes, dark leafy veggies, etcup

Oleic acid – This ingredient is what has omega 9 fatty acids. You can find it in virgin olive oil.

Curcumin – This is very powerful and is found in turmeric powder, which is a spice.

Alpha-lipoic acid - This is an antioxidant and comes in many kinds of products like meats and veggies, but you can also take it as a supplement.

Some Possible Challenges That Can Occur with the Anti-Inflammatory Diet

One thing about the Anti-Inflammatory Diet is that it may promote too much salt in the diet as a sample menu showed an average of more than 3,300 mg of salt, while normal dietary guidelines say we should not have more than about half that much every day. Plus, dietary guidelines say we should get more than 4,000 mg of potassium a day and a typical daily menu from the anti-inflammatory diet showed around 1,500 mg a day. However, it is very hard to get enough potassium in a normal diet, as not many foods provide a lot of it.

It is someone lacking in calcium as well, with an average daily amount of around 800mg, whereas the government guidelines say

Robert Wilson

we should get around 1,300 day, depending on the person, as some women should have even more calcium if she is pregnant or nursing.

Vitamin D is also lacking in the anti-inflammatory diet and the daily average menu showed no vitamin D. This is bad as we should be getting around 15 micrograms a day, especially if you live in an area that doesn't get much sunlight.

All in all, if you want to get rid of inflammation in the body, following this diet can help you to do that and possibly help you to fight off obesity and certain kinds of illnesses.

CHAPTER 2- WHAT ARE THE SYMPTOMS OF FOOD ALLERGIES AND THE ANTI-INFLAMMATION DISEASE?

Food allergy is an extremely common problem that affects almost all people at one point or the other. Similar sentiments can be said about the common problem of food intolerance. Despite the predominant cases of allergic reaction to food and food intolerance, research studies have indicated that only about 6 to 8% of children and 3% of adults have medically proven true food allergy and reaction. Indeed in the United States up to 15 million individuals are affected by the problem of food allergy, this includes 1 in 3 children.

The existing disparity between instances of food intolerance, which is often mistaken for food allergy, and clinically proven food allergies is as a result of widespread public perception and misinterpretation that any reaction that leads to food intolerance is labeled as food allergy. Food intolerance is usually a much more common problem than that of food allergy.

The Symptoms of Food Allergies

The problem of food allergy is growing and can get critical if the causes are not dealt with at the opportune time. It is imperative to note that the problem of food allergy in children is acutely different from that which afflicts the adults. The problem is aggravated because it is much easier for children to overcome the problem of food allergies than their adult counterparts. The problem of food allergy specifically concerns food and dietary choices, food allergy can be easily treated by avoiding the specific food diets that are known to exacerbate the problem. Medics can diagnosis the problem of food allergy after studying the patient history and diet.

Robert Wilson

True food allergy can be described as an abnormal response to food, and it is usually elicited by a certain reaction in the body's immunity, the immune system is vital in identifying and destroying germs that cause disease. Food allergy comes about when the body's immune system targets the body's harmless food protein. Usually the allergen components in food are responsible for triggering the allergic reactions, food allergy and reaction may manifest itself in many ways. To some people this reaction may be life threatening and a frightening experience, but to some, food allergy reaction may only result in non threatening responses such as restlessness. The most common symptoms of food allergy are:

- ➤ Fainting and dizziness
- ➤ Trouble breathing and wheezing
- ➤ Itching of the mouth or tingling
- ➤ Vomiting, diarrhea and abdominal pain
- ➤ Eczema, hives and itching sometimes uncomfortable
- ➤ Difficulty swallowing
- ➤ Drop in blood pressure
- ➤ Unexplained rapid pulse rate

The symptoms of food allergy are usually evident in many parts of the body; these symptoms can affect the skin, digestive system and the respiratory system. The symptoms that affect the body's largest organ, the skin and can manifest in welts, itching, atopic dermatitis, redness and swelling. These symptoms are, however, more pronounced and common to children. The symptoms of food allergy in the digestive system include stomach cramps, throat and mouth itching, nausea, and rectal bleeding especially in children.

The symptoms in the respiratory system include wheezing, running nose and difficulty breathing. Children may specifically exhibit symptoms such as eczema, wheezing and running nose when experiencing soy or milk induced allergies. However, extreme symptoms may include colic, severe diarrhea, poor growth and constipation.

Anti-Inflammation Diseases and Conditions

Food allergy can lead to severe reactions that can generate to conditions such as anaphylaxis. Anaphylaxis is a fatal, and life threatening condition that can cause death or coma if left untreated or not treated on time. The symptoms of anaphylaxis include reduction in blood pressure leading to shock, lightheadedness and loss of consciousness, tightening of airways and constriction, high pulse rate, difficulty breathing and swelling of the throat. Anaphylaxis can manifest itself within minutes or it may occur and re-occur after few hours of eating food; the other triggers for anaphylaxis include seafood, peanuts, alcohol, and Aspirin.

The other common factors that can lead to food allergy include exercise and pollen triggers. The exercise induced food allergy affects many people who do regular exercises, the symptoms usually appear as soon as one begins exercising. These symptoms include lightheadedness (fainting) and itchiness; the causes are usually as a result of an eaten substance. The pollen food allergy is also known as the oral allergy syndrome and is normally triggered after taking certain nuts, spices, fresh fruits or vegetables.

The protein ingredient in vegetables and fruits can lead to reactions similar to reactions that are caused by the body's inbuilt response to certain pollens. Both the pollen and exercise induced allergies can lead to anaphylaxis if not treated on time. Research studies are ongoing to look into the effects of heredity as a trigger for food allergy, especially where both or one of the parents is allergic to certain foods.

Robert Wilson

It is incumbent upon individuals who are afflicted with food allergy, to see an allergist or consult a doctor if they notice any such symptoms immediately after taking a meal. Seeking immediate medical assistance can also help reduce severe cases of food allergy such as anaphylaxis. Other classified causes of allergy include severe colds, toxins reaction cigarette smoking, stress, inflammatory bowel disease and food poisoning. Most doctors prescribe epinephrine to manage and treat the anaphylaxis condition. The treatment requires that the patient learn how to use the auto-injector. The epinephrine prescription usually expires within 1 year as such it is essential for the users of this drug to check the expiry dates and renew their prescriptions in time.

The best way to manage anti-inflammatory conditions and diseases is by reducing or eliminating foods that promote inflammation; this can go a long way in reducing the cases of inflammation since food allergy and intolerance are a common acknowledge problem. The foods that promote inflammation include trans-fats, refined carbohydrates, saturated fats, corn and soybean oil, dairy, red meat and sugars. On the hand, foods that are known to possess anti-inflammatory benefits include ginger, blueberries, turmeric, green tea, olive oil and cherries. Such provisions should be introduced in the diet or be encouraged depending on the need and doctors advice.

CHAPTER 3- WHY IS AN ANTI-INFLAMMATION DIET IMPORTANT?

As mentioned in previous chapters, the anti-inflammation diet is very important to your overall health because it has so many long lasting benefits. When you can limit or eliminate the foods in your diet that cause inflammation, your body can benefit in many more ways than simply losing weight. Chronic inflammation will continue to occur within the body as long as certain foods are digested, and those foods do have the potential to lead to other diseases like heart disease or heart failure. In this chapter we will discuss some of the common foods that cause the inflammation within the body and the benefits to eliminating them from your diet.

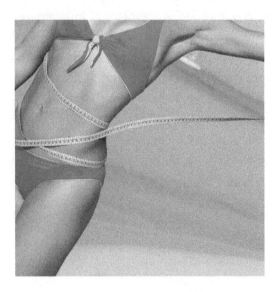

Losing Weight with the Anti-Inflammation Diet

When you can eliminate those foods that are causing you pain within the body, you are left to better enjoy foods that are much better for you health wise. Milk, eggs, and certain meats that cause inflammation can also be the cause of your weight gain as well.

Take the time to look for the foods that will not affect your body any further with inflammation and can help you to promote a healthier lifestyle. Once you condition your body to enjoy the new foods, you will see how your metabolism works much more efficiently at removing any fatty deposits in the blood stream. When the body can cleanse itself easier the deposits that cause fat to build up will have a much harder time.

When you feel less pain from the foods that you eat and you see your body beginning to transform, your emotional state ill change for the better as well. When you are always in pain your brain uses food as a mechanism to try and eliminate the pain. The brain thinks because you crave certain foods, that by getting you to eat them, the craving will be abated. What happens is you get on an endless treadmill of eating and pain that can often lead to serious diseases within the body. Enjoying your new anti-inflammation diet will help you mentally as well as physically.

Increased Energy with the Anti-Inflammation Diet

Most foods that cause inflammation within the body are full of sugars and flours that give you a quick burst of energy, to only leave you feeling lethargic and sluggish a few hours later. When the foods that cause you pain drain your energy, they also have a negative impact on your mental health as well. When you eat these foods for lunch you may get a quick burst that helps you during the next hours at work.

Suddenly the chronic pain sets in and that energy boost is long gone. Besides feeling sluggish, you now have to deal with a brain that is having difficulty focusing on the task at hand. The ability to think clearly and concentrate has been washed away with your energy, and you find yourself grabbing something to give you that burst to make it through the day. This is not only unhealthy for your body, it can do harm to your mental health as well.

An anti-inflammation diet will allow you to eat foods that not only give you that burst of energy; they can keep you alert through the afternoon without any pain within your body. Foods like raw fruits and vegetables will not cause your body any pain and contain enough nutrients to keep you alert and energized through the afternoon. Keeping a bowl of grapes or fresh carrots near your desk will help you to feed any hunger cravings throughout the day, while helping you to avoid the physical and mental pain of those sugary foods that only spike your levels short term. When you change your diet to contain more foods high in polyphenols, you can sustain your energy levels to get you through the entire afternoon. With fewer cravings for sugar and fewer mental crashes each day, your body benefits from a more peak physical condition as well as staying mentally alert.

Preventing Chronic Diseases with an Anti-Inflammation Diet

Chronic diseases can be significantly reduced when you implement an anti-inflammation diet into your routine. These diseases can range from rheumatoid arthritis, heart disease, allergies, Crohn's disease, psoriasis, and ulcerative colitis. These foods that have been causing you chronic pain also have the ability to age the body faster. The skin will appear much older looking and your organs will show to be years beyond their age when you continue eating foods that cause inflammation. A simple switch to a more nutritional diet can help prevent chronic diseases from forming in the first place.

The most effective way to reduce chronic diseases from the body is a combination of a healthy diet, anti-inflammatory lifestyle, and exercise. This is the most natural way to cure the body from within and can help you to better manage those conditions that occur once the food has activated the inflammation. There have been many studies recently released that show that an anti-inflammation diet can have a direct impact on metabolic syndrome. These biomarkers have a direct association with diabetes and heart disease. The study went on to show that patients who participated in the study showed a significant decrease in metabolic syndrome from 44% to an amazing 24%. This drop took place in an amazingly short 8 weeks.

Enjoying Your Food with an Anti-Inflammation Diet

The biggest problem with most of the diets on the market today is that they continue to remind you of the foods you crave. When you new diet claims that they have a pizza, cookies, or cakes that are created with better ingredients, you simply get reminded of those delicious foods that are causing inflammation in your body. When you start your new anti-inflammation diet, you can create an entirely new variety of foods that you can fall in love with that are actually good for you. This way you aren't reminded of those chocolate éclairs, chocolate chip cookies, and deep dish pizzas.

Create a new menu in your home that is rich in fish, chicken, and turkey. Create dishes that will keep you healthy and that you enjoy eating too. These changes will be challenging at first, but they will reduce the inflammation and improve your physical and mental health for the long term.

CHAPTER 4- USEFUL INGREDIENTS AND KITCHEN UTENSILS TO HAVE WHEN PREPARING ANTI-INFLAMMATION DIET RECIPES

One of the great things about starting an anti-inflammation diet is that it is not overly complex. You can probably begin switching to an anti-inflammation diet without making any drastic changes to your kitchen or buying specialty products. However, there are some items that you will eventually see as indispensable if you continue the anti-inflammation lifestyle. Below is a list of kitchen gadgets you might want to acquire, followed by some basic food-items you should keep your pantry stocked with.

KITCHEN GADGETS

A Good Fillet Knife

One major component of the anti-inflammation diet is increasing your intake of Omega-3 fatty acids, such as those found in fish. Unfortunately, the practice of preparing fresh fish seems to be a dying art in American homes. To make the preparation of fish less intimidating and more fun you should make sure you have an appropriate fillet knife, and know how to use it. An all-purpose fillet knife with a blade around seven inches, and a rubber handle should be adequate for preparing most fatty fishes.

A Water Filter

Cutting out the sugary drinks is a large part of an anti-inflammation diet. However, just because you are cutting back on cola does not mean you should reduce your fluid intake. You should still be drinking at least eight glasses of water each day. A great way to improve the taste of your water, and make sure you are drinking it, is to invest in a quality water filter. You can look into filters that attach directly to your faucet, or purchase a specialized water pitcher with a filter. Alternatively, you can purchase purified water from the store. Unfortunately with that option, many people simply stop drinking enough water when they forget to purchase more.

A Tea Infuser

Another good way to increase your fluid intake while avoiding sugary, processed drinks is to start drinking teas and herbal infusions. A tea infuser, which you can fill with fresh herbs from your garden, allows you to enjoy hot and cold beverages with varying flavors. Additionally, many herbs such as ginger or chamomile have anti-inflammatory properties.

A Nut Cracker

Nuts are high in vitamins, minerals, and healthy fats. However, you might want to buy fresh nuts that are neither roasted nor salted to get the most benefits. To enjoy these nuts make sure you have a strong cracker at home that will not tire your hands.

A Rice Cooker

Rice cookers are not just for cooking rice. You can effectively cook any whole grain in a rice cooker, saving time and electricity, and freeing up your stove for other things. A great thing about whole grains is that they keep well for 2-3 days after they are cooked, so you can feel free to make a large batch in your rice cooker to eat as a side dish for several days.

BASIC FOODS

Vegetables

It is true that vegetables will not last in your kitchen for an entire month, and yet many Americans only shop once or twice a month. You should go shopping for fresh vegetables every week, and make sure you stock up on peppers, and tomatoes, two of the most useful vegetables in an anti-inflammatory diet. Also, get plenty of leafy greens such as spinach and chard when they are in season. Although you can purchase canned tomatoes and peppers make sure you read the ingredients and avoid canned products that are high in salt. If you have the opportunity it is always better to shop often and go fresh with your produce.

Fruits and Berries

While it is good to increase your overall fruit intake, it is especially good to look for bright red fruits and berries such as red raspberries and sour cherries. These fruits are high in antioxidants and low in calories. As an added bonus, if you are able to grow a red raspberry plant in your garden, you can use the leaves to make a healthy, anti-oxidant tea.

Ginger and Turmeric

These two spices can add a lot of flavor to your cooking. Research has not yet shown how effective these two roots are in battling inflammation, but they certainly will not hurt. Ginger can be eaten raw, added to meals, or infused into a tea. Turmeric makes excellent curries and stews filled with color and flavor. If possible you should buy these in their root form and grate them as needed, but you can also purchase them as dried powders.

Garlic and Onions

Garlic and onions contain many anti-inflammatory chemicals that work similarly to the chemicals used in pain-reduction medication. They also keep for quite a bit longer than other fruits and vegetables and are easy to grow if you want to keep your own home supply.

Olive Oil

Use olive oil instead of vegetable oil on salads and when cooking at low temperatures, such as roasting peppers or tomatoes. Cooking at high temperatures with olive oil is a debated topic. Generally, as long as the oil is not heated to the point of smoking it is still safe to consume. However, many people find it tastes better when cooked at low temperatures. Make sure you purchase virgin, cold-pressed olive oil for the most benefits. Olive oil will generally keep for up to a year so you do not have to worry about it spoiling if you decide to buy it in bulk.

Whole Grains

Replace your processed grains with whole grains. You should keep a stock of brown rice, bulgur, quinoa, and oats in your pantry. Many processed foods claim to be, "whole grain," and while they do contain some whole grains they also often contain processed grains and sugars that are not necessary for your diet. By having pure whole grains at home to cook with you can avoid the trap of "whole grain," packaging altogether.

From these lists you can see that following an anti-inflammation diet does not require many specialty items or ingredients. Ultimately it is about choosing fresh, unprocessed foods which you can prepare any way you like. However, these items may help to inspire you and keep you going on a healthy, anti-inflammation diet.

CHAPTER 5- SOME SAMPLE MENUS OR MEAL PLANS FOR ANTI-INFLAMMATION DIET

Because of the many health benefits that can be obtained by making changes in diet, many people have decided to give the anti-inflammation diet a try. It has been proven that inflammation is the principal cause of many diseases such as rheumatoid arthritis. Many people that suffer from this disease have decided to make big changes in the way that they eat in order to avoid the effects of inflammation pain. Even those people that do not suffer from any inflammation disease could really benefit from this diet as well.

There are many delicious recipes that one could make using the base foods from this diet as a way to plan out the meals for their day. While there are many different foods that are allowed in the diet, there are some fruits, vegetables, meats and oils that really stand out as great foods for fighting off inflammation. The following is a list of those foods.

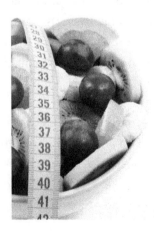

Tart Cherries- Tart cherries are an amazing fruit. They have super high red pigment and the properties that are found in this fruit have been proven to reduce inflammation. Experts say that this anti-oxidant fruit has the highest ant-inflammatory content found in any fruit.

Berries- Berries are an excellent snack and they also make great compliments to any meal. Berries are very low in calories and they are great for maintaining inflammation at bay.

Olive Oil- Olive oil is a very heart healthy oil. Any food that is part of the heart healthy diet is also great for the anti-inflammation diet as well.

Garlic and Onions- These two vegetables are amazing for their work against inflammation, because of the chemicals that are found in both of these vegetables. These chemicals work directly in the body to fight against inflammation.

Beets- These vegetables are very rich in red pigmentation. They have wonderful properties in them that not only have been proven to reduce inflammation in the body, but they have also been proven to reduce the risk of cancer and many other diseases.

Soy- Soy has chemicals that are called Isoflavones. Isoflavones help reduce inflammation, so it is a great idea to substitute tofu for meat a few times a week.

Dark Leafy Greens- Dark leafy greens like spinach, broccoli and kale have wonderful properties that aid in anti-inflammatory action.

Whole Grains- Many studies have been done that prove that foods that are whole grains can aid in lowering inflammation. It is a good idea to replace foods like white bread and white rice with whole grains instead.

Fatty Fish- Fatty fish are very rich in omega-3 oils. Omega 3 has natural properties that help reduce inflammation. It is not all fish, but Salmon and Mackerel are two of the best fish that are rich in healthy fats.

Nuts- All nuts have anti-oxidant properties and these can help fight off and repair any damage that is caused by inflammation. In particular almonds are great because they are also very high in fiber.

With these foods in mind it is easy to get a nice meal plan for a person or for a family. A great meal plan might look something like one of the following

Meal Plan #1

Breakfast

Low fat yogurt with honey, almonds and raspberries and a cup of green tea

Lunch

A whole wheat bread salmon sandwich; the salmon can be cooked with an apricot glaze and then placed on wheat bread. Add spinach, tomato, feta cheese and a little bit of olive oil to the sandwich. Whole wheat crackers can be had as a side snack, and a half a cup of cherries.

Snack

A half of a cup of mixed nuts

Dinner

Garlic Chicken with Whole Grain Brown Rice

Robert Wilson
Ingredients

Garlic Chicken
¼ cup of garlic
¼ cup of onions
2 teaspoons of olive oil
½ pound of chopped chicken
½ cup of chicken broth
½ teaspoon of ginger
1 teaspoon of garlic powder

Directions

Sauté the garlic and the onion together until the onion runs clear. Next add the chicken until it is fully cooked. Next add the chicken broth and then the rest of the ingredients. Cook for another fifteen minutes and then serve over brown rice.

Dessert

A cup of mixed berries, walnuts, with a whipped cream topping

Snack

An organic apple and 1 table spoon of peanut butter.

Meal Plan #2

Breakfast

Healthy green shake with almonds

Green shake

Ingredients

1 cup of kale
1 cup of spinach
½ an apple
¼ cup of apple juice

Directions

Use a blender to blend all of the ingredients in the shake together.

Lunch

Green Salad (however you wish to mix it) with beats, salmon, and feta cheese. Have an oil and vinegar dressing and a fruit cocktail for the dessert.

Snack

An organic apple and ¼ cup of walnuts

Dinner

Tofu and stir fried vegetables over brown rice.

Ingredients

1 bag of mixed stir vegetables for stir fry
½ pound of cut tofu
1 teaspoon of olive oil
¼ cup of soy sauce
2 eggs
½ tablespoon of ginger

Directions

Stir fry the vegetables on the stove with the olive oil for about five to ten minute or until the vegetables are almost soft. Once they are almost soft then add the two eggs and scramble them with the vegetables. Next add the ginger and the soy sauce and cook for about ten more minutes. Serve stir fry over brown rice

Dessert

Fruit salad (any mixed fruit)

Snack

A handful of almonds

Eating the anti-inflammation diet is not as hard as it may sound. It just involves making a few small changes in diet. The foods that are recommended are foods that are rich in nutrients, anti-oxidants, and vitamins. This is a good diet for anyone to consider taking up especially if a person is suffering from any type of inflammatory disease, autoimmune disease, or joint disease. People take different medications in order to help them reduce pain and inflammation. It is good to know that just a few small changes in the diet can make a world of difference. There have been accounts of people that have even gone off their anti-inflammation medication. It is really worth the effort to investigate this diet, because it could change a person's entire life and their health for the better.

CHAPTER 6- 8 ANTI-INFLAMMATION DIET APPETIZER RECIPES

Sesame Seared Tuna Bites

Ingredients

1.5 pounds sushi grade tuna
2 tablespoon course ground pepper
2 tablespoon course ground sea salt
 2 tablespoon black sesame seeds
2 tablespoon white sesame seeds
1 tablespoon sesame oil
2 tablespoon canola oil

Directions

Mix together pepper, salt and seeds in a shallow bowl. Tuna steak should be about 1 to 1.5-inch thick. Trim the skin and cut into triangles of equal size. Press sides of each triangle into seed mixture and place on a flat surface covered with parchment. Mix oils together and heat in a large, flat frying pan until it begins to smoke. You will want to maintain this high heat throughout the cooking process. Place about 6 triangles in the pan, seed side down, about 10 seconds, and then turn each onto another side. When all three sides have been seared, remove and place on a paper towel to drain. Arrange seared tuna bites onto a serving plate, cover with plastic and refrigerate until cool. Serve with soy sauce mixed with equal amounts of minced ginger and garlicup

Rosemary Marcona Almonds

Ingredients

Robert Wilson

1 pound Marcona almonds, toasted
Olive oil
2-3 sprigs of fresh rosemary or a few pinches of dried rosemary
Coarse ground sea salt

Directions

Mix oil, rosemary and salt in a large bowl. Add almonds and stir until evenly coated. Store the almonds in an airtight container until ready to serve.

Edamame Appetizer

These are eaten holding the pod by the stem and sliding the beans out with your teeth. Discard the pod.

Ingredients

1 pound fresh edamame, in the pod
Coarse ground sea salt

Directions

Bring a large pot of water to boil. Add edamame and boil until tender but crisp, about 7-10 minutes. Start checking for doneness at about 7 minutes. When satisfied with doneness run under cold water to stop cooking. Drain and pat off extra moisture with a paper towel. Sprinkle with enough salt to taste.

Roasted Red Pepper Dip

This dip can be used as a dip, a spread for sandwiches or served as a condiment with meat and vegetables.

Ingredients

1 cup plain, non-fat Greek yogurt

½ cup finely chopped roasted red peppers

1 tablespoon olive oil

1 tablespoon lemon juice

1 clove garlic, minced

Salt and pepper to taste

Directions

Mix all ingredients in a bowl until well blended. Refrigerate until ready to serve.

Beet and Feta Bruschetta

These are colorful and full of flavor.

Ingredients

2 beets (try to use a variety of colors)

Feta cheese

Slices of whole grain baguette

Olive oil

1 clove garlic (cut in half)

Fresh mint, chopped (optional)

Directions

Slice the beets, half the slices, then grill or roast in the oven until tender. Check for tenderness by using a fork. If a fork passes easily through the beets they are done.

Grill or toast slices of bread until just turning brown. Rub one side of each bread slice with garlic then drizzle with oil.

Place 2-3 slices of beet on each piece of bread. Sprinkle with feta and top with just a bit of mint.

Robert Wilson
Turmeric Veggie Appetizer

This can also be used as a dip for other vegetables (carrots, celery, peppers, etc.).

Ingredients

1 cup soaked cashews
1 cup young coconut flesh
¼ cup water from the coconut
2 tablespoon olive oil
1 clove garlic
2 tsp. turmeric
1 tsp. fresh, minced ginger root
2 tablespoon agave
1 sliced cucumber

Directions

Process all ingredients in a food processor until smooth, scraping down the sides frequently. Slice cucumbers into rounds, not too thin. Pipe the dip onto the middle of each round and garnish with a little paprika.

Onion & Garlic Dip

This is so much better than store bought.

Ingredients

1 large onion, finely chopped
4-6 cloves garlic, minced
1 tablespoon extra-virgin olive oil
1 16 oz. low fat sour cream
Juice of 1 lemon

2 tsp. hot pepper sauce
1 tsp. paprika
Salt to taste

Directions

Heat oil in heavy skillet over medium-high heat, sauté onions and garlic until soft and then blend in food processor with remaining ingredients until mostly smooth. Refrigerate until ready to serve.

Berry-Stuffed Portobello

These can also be served as the main dish for a luncheon.

Ingredients

4 large Portobello mushrooms, each about 4 inches across
1 tablespoon extra virgin olive oil
4-5 asparagus trimmed and cut into 1-inch pieces
1/3 cup red pepper, finely chopped
1 small green onion or shallot, finely chopped
2 tsp. oregano
1 tsp. salt
¼ tsp. black pepper
1 cup raspberries and/or blueberries
4 oz. crumbled tomato basil feta cheese
½ cup toasted walnuts, chopped

Directions

Line a broiler pan with aluminum foil. Remove mushroom stems and gills, discard. Rub some of the oil on both sides of the remaining caps and season with salt and pepper. Place caps, gill-side down, on prepared pan and broil 4-5 minutes. Remove and set aside.

Robert Wilson

Heat the oven to 350F. Combine remaining ingredients in microwave-safe bowl until well blended. Microwave at 50% for 3-5 minutes and stir once or twice during cooking. Scoop equally into mushroom caps and return pan to preheated oven. Bake 25-30 minutes or until mushrooms are tender. Drizzle with balsamic vinegar (optional).

CHAPTER 7- 8 ANTI-INFLAMMATION DIET LUNCH RECIPES

Arthritis is a painful malady which has no cure. The most any sufferer can hope for is to get some relief through diet and medication. Check out these recipes to help you enjoy a lunch that will also help reduce the inflammation in your joints.

Sweet Potato and Black Bean Burgers with Lime Mayonnaise

The foods to fight arthritis in this recipe are the sweet potatoes and the garlic.

Ingredients

½ cup mayonnaise (reduced or low fat)
1 lime
½ teaspoon hot sauce
Cooking spray
1 small chopped onion
1 minced jalapeno
2 teaspoons ground cumin
2 teaspoons minced garlic
2 cans drained and mashed black beans (14.5 ounces each)
2 cups raw sweet potato, grated
1 lightly beaten egg
1 cup breadcrumbs divided
Hamburger buns

Directions

Begin by preheating your broiler to medium-high. The oven rack will need to be four or five inches from the broiler. Zest the lime into a bowl and add mayonnaise and hot sauce. Stir those together then refrigerate the mixture. Spray a large skillet with the cooking spray then heat it to medium-high. Add the onions and cook them until they're tender. Mix in the jalapeno, garlic and cumin then cook for only half a minute. Move the onion mixture from the heat to a bowl and add the sweet potato, black beans, half cup breadcrumbs and egg. Combine all of this together. Take this mixture and form it into eight patties. Sprinkle the other half of the breadcrumbs over the burgers, which you've already placed on a greased baking pan. Broil the patties for eight to ten minutes on each side or until they are a toasty brown. Serve with the mayonnaise in the refrigerator.

Pumpkin Soup

The arthritis fighters in this soup are the pumpkin, ginger and garlic.

Ingredients

1 cup chopped onion
1 inch peeled and minced gingerroot
1 clove minced garlic
6 cups vegetable stock
4 cups pureed pumpkin
1 teaspoon salt
½ teaspoon chopped thyme
½ cup half-and-half
1 one teaspoon chopped parsley

Directions

Place a large pot on the heat. Heat it to medium-high. It's going to be a larger sized pot for this recipe. Cook the garlic, onions and ginger in approximately a half cup of the vegetable stock. It will get tender in about five minutes. Add the pumpkin, the rest of the vegetable stock, the thyme and salt. Cook this for thirty minutes. Grab the handheld blender and mix up the soup until it's a smooth consistency. Take the soup off the stove and mix in the half-and-half. Sprinkle parsley on the top.

Kippers Salad

The good stuff in this recipe are the kippers and the garlic.

Ingredients

½ cup mayonnaise
1 finely chopped
Small onion
1 finely chopped stalk of celery
1 tablespoon chopped parsley
1 teaspoon of lemon juice
1 minced garlic clove
⅛ an eighth teaspoon of both salt and pepper
6 ounce can of drained kippers.

Directions

Use a medium bowl to mix up all ingredients except the kippers. Add the kippers and toss it all together gently to mix it all up. Refrigerate it until you're ready to eat it.

Roasted Chicken Wraps

The red cabbage is the main arthritis fighter here.

Ingredients

½ cup mayonnaise
2 tablespoons of pickle juice
1 teaspoon black pepper

Robert Wilson
1½ cups red cabbage, shredded
1 tablespoon of apple cider vinegar
¼ teaspoon salt
¼ teaspoon cayenne pepper
1 roasted, cooled chicken
6 flatbreads

Directions

Begin by combining the pickle juice, mayonnaise and pepper into a bowl. Put that in the refrigerator. Use another bowl to combine vinegar, cabbage, cayenne pepper and salt. Toss it lightly to mix it together. Shred the chicken into small pieces, adding the pieces to the mayonnaise mixture in the refrigerator. Split the cabbage and chicken mixes evenly among the flatbreads, roll and enjoy.

Persimmon and Pear Salad

The super foods here are the persimmons, olive oil, spinach and garlic.

Ingredients

1 teaspoon mustard
2 tablespoons lemon juice
3 tablespoons olive oil
1 minced shallot
1 teaspoon of minced garlic
1 sliced ripe persimmon
1 sliced red pear
½ cup toasted chopped pecans
6 cups of baby spinach

Directions

Combine the mustard, lemon juice, olive oil, shallot and garlic into a salad bowl. Put in the rest of the ingredients and toss together. Serve right away.

Roasted Sweet Potato Soup

The foods to fight arthritis in this recipe are the sweet potatoes, ginger and orange juice.

Ingredients

2½ pounds of sweet potatoes
1 tablespoon olive oil
¼ teaspoon of both salt and pepper
1½ cups leeks, thinly sliced
1 inch of peeled, minced ginger
1 teaspoon of minced garlic
½ cup of dry white wine
1 teaspoon thyme leaves, chopped
5 cups of vegetable broth
2 cups of orange juice

Directions

Preheat the oven until it is four hundred degrees Fahrenheit. Cut the potatoes into small pieces, approximately one inch. Toss them together with olive oil, pepper and salt and put them on a baking pan. Put them in the oven, roasting them for up to fifty minutes until they are tender. Stir them a few times while they cook. Use a soup pot or Dutch oven, coated with cooking spray, to cook the leeks in medium-high heat. They need to be tender and wilted. It will take approximately eight minutes. Mix in the ginger and the garlic, cooking for one minute. Put in the wine and let it boil. This will cook until all the wine evaporates. Add the broth. Mix in the sweet potato and thyme mixture then boil again. Reduce the heat

Robert Wilson

and let it cook until everything is tender. Puree this mix in small batches.

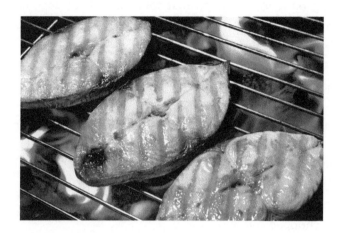

Smoked Trout Tartine

The good foods in this recipe are red peppers, trout, olive oil, lemon and cannellini beans.

Ingredients

2 tablespoons lemon juice
1 tablespoon olive oil
1 teaspoon mustard
A pinch of sugar
¾ pounds flaked smoked trout
2 tablespoons rinsed and drained capers
½ cup roasted, diced red peppers
½ can cannellini beans (15 ounces), drained and rinsed
1 stalk of finely chopped celery
2 tablespoons of minced onion
1 teaspoon of chopped dill
4 large toasted bread slices
Dill for a garnish

Directions

Use a big bowl to whisk the first four ingredients together. Add everything else except the bread and toss it all together. Add the mixture to one slice of bread and garnish with the dill sprig.

Lentil and Garbanzo Soup

The turmeric and ginger in this recipe help fight inflammation.

Ingredients

2 chopped onions
1 cup of chopped celery
1 cup of diced carrots
2 teaspoons ginger, grated
1 teaspoon garlic, minced
1 teaspoon garam masala
1 teaspoon turmeric
½ teaspoon ground cumin
¼ teaspoon cayenne pepper, ground
6 cups of vegetable stock
1 cup of lentils
2 cans drained and rinsed garbanzo beans (15 ounce)
1 can undrained petite tomatoes (14.5 ounces)

Directions

In a large pot coated with some cooking spray heated to medium-high, saute the onions until they're tender. Add the celery and carrots then cook for five more minutes. Mix in the garlic, garam masala, turmeric, cumin and cayenne pepper and simmer for half a minute. Add the broth with all the other ingredients then cook it until the lentils feel tender. It will take about an hour and a half.

CHAPTER 8- 8 ANTI-INFLAMMATION DIET DINNER RECIPES

Turkey with Chili

Ingredients

1 tablespoon minced garlic
1 large onion, chopped
1½ pounds turkey (ground)
2 cups water
2 tablespoons chili powder
1 can drained and rinsed kidney beans (16-ounce)
1 (28-ounce) can canned crushed tomatoes
1 teaspoon oregano (dried)
1 teaspoon hot sauce
1 teaspoon smoked paprika
1 teaspoon cumin (ground)
2 teaspoons turmeric

Directions

Spray a big pot with cooking oil, let onions cook until tender, for about 5 min until they are a brownish color. Put in garlic and cook for half a minute. Put in the turkey and combine until cooked. After 10 minutes of stirring add the remaining ingredients and water and let come to a boil.

After boiling let it simmer for 30-45 min.

Brazil Nut-Crusted Tilapia with Sautéed Kale

Ingredients

2 tablespoons sesame seeds (toasted)

¼ teaspoon kosher salt

1½ heads chopped kale

1 clove mashed garlic

1 tablespoon sesame oil

Vegetable cooking spray

1½ pounds tilapia fillets

¼ cup whole grain mustard

2 tablespoons grated Parmesan cheese

½ cup fresh bread crumbs

¼ cup Brazil nuts (roasted)

Directions

Preheat the oven to 400°F. Grease the baking sheet then put it to one side.

Put the Brazil nuts in blender and pulse mix in the Parmesan cheese and breadcrumbs.

Place tilapia fillets on the baking sheet that was set aside and spread with the mustard. Spread Brazil nut mix lightly over the tilapia and spray breadcrumbs lightly with the cooking spray. Bake for no more than 10 minutes (until the tilapia is cooked through).

Heat a big skillet over medium-high heat. Put in the sesame oil let it heat before putting in the garlic (approx. 15 seconds). After another 15 seconds put in the chopped kale. Stir frequently until kale is tender (approximately 7 minutes). Combine with sesame seed

Serve fish at once with a side of kale.

Red Pepper and Turkey Pasta

Robert Wilson

Ingredients

2 pounds hot, cooked protein-rich rigatoni
2 pounds turkey (ground)
1 tablespoon red wine vinegar
2 tablespoons chopped fresh oregano
2 teaspoons garlic (minced)
1 large chopped onion
3 tablespoons extra virgin olive oil
3 large red bell peppers

Directions

Coarsely chop peppers and take out the stem and seeds.

Heat oil then put in the onion and peppers and cook until tender (20 minutes), then add garlic.

Puree this mixture until smooth in a blender. Reheat sauce on medium-low heat. Mix in the vinegar and oregano and fine-tune seasonings.

Spray e skillet with cooking oil and sauté turkey until cooked and brownish. Put the turkey in the sauce and let simmer for 20 minutes.

Add cooked turkey to sauce and simmer to perfection. Serve with hot pasta.

Steamed Salmon with Lemon Scented Zucchini

Ingredients

¼ teaspoon pepper (freshly ground)
¼ teaspoon kosher salt
4 (6-ounce) salmon fillets

½ cup water
1 cup white wine
2 small thinly sliced zucchini
1 thinly sliced lemon
1 thinly sliced onion

Directions

Put the water, white wine, zucchini, lemon and onion in a Dutch oven let steam. Place over medium-high heat until liquid starts to boil.

Season the fish with pepper and salt. Lower heat and gently place the fish on the rack over the steaming vegetables. Cover and let steam until thoroughly cooked.

Serve fish on a bed of vegetables. Top with the sliced olives. Garnish if desired.

Sweet Potato and Black Bean Burgers with Lime Mayonnaise

Ingredients

Whole wheat hamburger buns
1 cup plain breadcrumbs, divided
1 lightly beaten egg
2 cups raw sweet potato (grated)
2 cans drained, rinsed and mashed black beans (14.5-ounce)
2 teaspoons garlic (minced)
2 teaspoons cumin (ground)
1 minced jalapeno
1 small chopped onion
Vegetable cooking spray
½ teaspoon hot sauce
1 lime

Robert Wilson
½ cup mayonnaise (reduced fat)

Directions

Preheat the grill or broiler for medium-high heat. Squeeze the lime into a bowl. Combine the hot sauce and mayonnaise. Refrigerate until ready to serve.

Spray a skillet with cooking oil and place over medium heat. Cook the onions for about 5 minutes until tender. Put in cumin and garlic jalapeno and cook for half a minute. Transfer onion mixture to a big bowl and combine ½ cup breadcrumbs, egg, sweet potato and mashed black beans.

Form eight patties from the mixture and sprinkle with the rest of the breadcrumbs. Place patties on a lightly greased baking sheet and spray evenly with cooking spray.

Broil until golden brown on each side (approximately 10 minutes). Serve at once on hamburger buns with lime mayonnaise.

Quinoa and Turkey Stuffed Peppers

Ingredients

3 red bell peppers
2 teaspoons fresh rosemary (chopped)
2 tablespoons fresh parsley (chopped)
3 tablespoons chopped toasted pecans
¼ cup extra-virgin olive oil
½ cup chicken stock
½ pound diced fully-cooked smoked turkey sausage
½ teaspoons salt
2 cups water
1 cup uncooked quinoa

Directions

Mix salt, water and quinoa in a big saucepan and let come to a boil. Turn down heat to low and then cover, and let simmer until all water is gone.

Remove the cover and leave for five minutes. Mix in rosemary, parsley, pecan, olive oil, chicken stock and sausage. Cut the peppers in half and remove the membranes and seeds. Cook for 5 minutes in boiling water and drain.

Put some of the quinoa mixture in each pepper and put it in a lightly greased baking dish (13-x 9-inch). Bake for 15 minutes at 350°F.

Roasted Chicken Wraps

Ingredients

6 mixed grain or whole wheat flatbreads
1 cooled deli-roasted chicken
¼ teaspoon cayenne pepper
¼ teaspoon kosher salt
1 tablespoon apple cider vinegar
1½ cups red cabbage (shredded)
1 teaspoon black pepper (freshly cracked)
2 tablespoons pickle juice

½ cup reduced-fat mayonnaise

Directions

Mix the pepper, pickle juice and mayonnaise in a big bowl and place in the refrigerator. In a bowl mix the cayenne pepper, salt, vinegar and cabbage. Cut the chicken into bite-sized pieces. Place the chicken in the mayonnaise mixture and combine well.

Divide cabbage and chicken mixtures evenly between the slices of flatbread and roll them.

Smoked Trout Tartine

Ingredients

4 large, ½-inch-thick toasted slices of crusty whole-grain bread
½ teaspoon dried or 1 teaspoon fresh dill (chopped)
2 tablespoons onion (minced)
1 stalk finely chopped celery
½ can drained and rinsed white kidney beans (cannellini beans) (15 ounce)
½ cup roasted red peppers (diced)
2 tablespoons rinsed and drained capers
¾ pound smoked trout (flake into bite-size pieces)
Pinch of sugar
1 teaspoon Dijon mustard
1 tablespoon extra-virgin olive oil
2 tablespoons lemon juice (freshly squeezed)
Dill sprigs (for garnish)

Directions

In a big bowl, mix sugar, Dijon mustard, olive oil and lemon juice.

Put in the rest of the ingredients except the bread. Place 1 slice of bread on a plate and spread the trout mixture on the top. Garnish if necessary.

ABOUT THE AUTHOR

Robert Wilson was not unfamiliar with the negative effects that arthritis can have on the individual as his mother has been battling with rheumatoid arthritis ever since she was in her thirties. He could see what the inflammation that is a direct result of the arthritis was doing to her. She never ever had any real relief until her doctor suggested that she try a particular diet to see if that would help reduce the level of inflammation.

As a result of this everybody had to go on this particular diet. He never had any issues with it as the food options were pleasing to the palate. From this experience, he made the decision to do a book that would not only help persons to understand the causes of inflammation but would also help them to learn which food combinations work best.